Solving The Neuropathy Puzzle

Cutting Edge Treatment
For Reversing Neuropathy

By Dr. Eric Auslander, D.C., B.C.N.

LEGAL NOTICES

The information contained in this book is based upon research and personal and professional experience of the author. It is not intended as a substitute for consulting with your healthcare provider. Any attempt to diagnose and treat an illness should be done under the direction of a healthcare professional.

The publisher and author do not advocate the use of any particular healthcare protocol, but believes the information in this book should be available to the public. The publisher and author are not responsible for any adverse effects or consequences resulting from the use of the suggestions, procedures, products and services discussed in this book. Should the reader have any questions concerning the appropriateness of any procedures or products mentioned, the author and publisher strongly suggest consulting with a professional healthcare advisor.

This is the United States of America and we as Americans shall be free to write and say whatever we choose. We respectfully request that you acknowledge that what is written in this book is protected by the First Amendment of the U.S. Constitution. If you cannot agree to the above, then please close this book and do not read any further. Your continued reading is your acknowledgement and agreement to hold harmless everyone from everything.

The information presented herein represents the view of the author as of the date of publication. Because of the rate with which conditions change, the author reserve the right to alter and update his opinion based on the new conditions. This book is for informational purposes only. While every attempt has been made to verify the information provided in this book, neither the authors nor their affiliates/partners assume any responsibility for errors, inaccuracies or omissions. Any slights of people or organizations are unintentional.

First Edition

Printed in the U.S.A.

ISBN: 9798687650717

Contents

About The Author

Dr. Eric Auslander is a Pittsburgh native. He received his Doctor of Chiropractic Degree from Life College, School of Chiropractic in Marietta Georgia and his Bachelor of Science degree from Arizona State University in Tempe Arizona.

He is licensed to practice chiropractic in Pennsylvania and South Carolina and is Board Certified by the National Board of Chiropractic Examiners. He also has an adjunctive license which allows him to render physiotherapy modalities.

Dr. Auslander has been awarded the Family Practice Award for Excellence in 2005, 2006, and 2007. He is a member of the Pennsylvania Chiropractic Association, International Chiropractic Pediatric Association, and Back Pack Safety America.

He is a Certified Chiropractic Insurance Consultant. He is certified in Peer Review and Independent Medical Examinations. Dr. Auslander is board certified in Neuropathy and Intractable Pain.

CHAPTER 1

Who's to Blame for America's Health Crisis?

People tend to think of today's health crisis in the United States as a health *insurance* crisis. Fingers have been pointed at many parties for the current state of affairs:

- Government, for the lack of universal and affordable health insurance.
- Pharmaceutical companies, for the ever-increasing price of prescription drugs.
- Health care industry, for poor managed health care practices.
- Food industry, because lower income individuals are practically forced to purchase cheap, highly processed, unhealthy foods.

Although each of these parties has a hand in perpetuating the crisis, none of them is the true cause. The real reason behind the health care crisis is each individual's poor choices and lifestyle, mostly in the areas of food, exercise, and stress management. This leads to health-related issues like cancer, heart disease, metabolic syndrome, stroke, diabetes, and so much more.

Whether we like it or not, each one of us must take personal responsibility for our health. This means educating ourselves about the choices that will make a positive change for us and for those we love.

Biggest Health Issue Is Big Indeed

Perhaps the biggest health issue in the United States is obesity. In fact, it is at epidemic proportions. Among Americans age 20 and older, 154.7 million are overweight or obese.

18% of deaths in America are associated with obesity. These deaths stem primarily from type 2 diabetes, hypertension, heart disease, liver disease, cancer, dementia, and depression.

How Did the Obesity Problem Get So Big?

Early in the 20th century, the American diet was quite different from what it is today. If you could hop in a time machine and peek onto the shelves at the local store your grandparents shopped at, you would find produce, living plants, seeds, and grains. You might also find some home canned products. You would not find today's grocery store travesties:

- Hormone injected meats
- Processed foods
- Fast foods
- Junk foods

With these "modern" food choices comes a completely different diet – the SAD diet (Standard American Diet). The foods found in the SAD diet are completely out of balance.

1. An excessive amount of meat, fats, and sugar
2. Too few fruits and vegetables
3. Lack of nutrients in the food due to overcooking and processing

Incredibly, billions of dollars have been spent on various studies in a quest to find the causes and solutions for obesity. But the real answer is sitting in plain sight in homes across America: specifically, in the kitchens and on the couches.

The answer to the obesity crisis, and the health care crisis in general, is simple – returning to a more natural diet rich in fresh fruits and vegetables, while avoiding processed foods, and being active every day.

Trying to Make the Perfect Food Better

Food companies work tirelessly at making the perfect foods – fruits, vegetables and grains – better by refining them and processing them and adding chemicals to them. Ironically, all this tinkering has created an American diet that is deficient.

Processed foods make up a huge percentage of the American diet. These food products are loaded with extra salt, sugar, artificial flavors, preservatives, and other chemicals. These foods are also missing vital nutrients and vitamins that are stripped away during processing. This adding and subtracting from our food is a recipe for disaster.

Whole, natural foods are perfect foods. Eating a wide variety of fruits, vegetables, and grains gives your body everything it needs for good health. The SAD diet does not.

What It Is and What It Isn't

The Standard American Diet, sadly, is high in calories and low in nutrition. It consists of foods such as:

- Refined flour
- Refined sugar
- Refined cooking oil
- Soft drinks
- Coffee
- Margarine
- Distilled liquor

In order to be healthy, we need to replace low nutrient foods with high nutrient, non-processed foods, including:

- Vegetables
- Fruits
- Lean meat in moderation
- Fish

A healthy body needs a diet high in vitamins, minerals, enzymes and antioxidants. It's the best way to make sure your body can correctly digest food, absorb nutrients, regulate cell function, and keep your body fueled up.

When your body doesn't have the nutrients it needs, the aging process speeds up. Aging doesn't just mean gray hair and wrinkles – we are talking about all the diseases associated with aging, such as:

- Coronary Heart Disease (CHD): About 600,000 people die of heart disease in the United States every year–that's 1 in every 4 deaths.

- Coronary heart disease alone costs the United States $108.9 billion each year.
- Stroke: In 2009, stroke caused 1 of every 19 deaths in the United States. On average, every 40 seconds, someone in the United States has a stroke. Every four minutes, someone dies from a stroke.
- High Blood Pressure: Based on data from 2007 to 2010, about 78 million people in the United States age 20 and older have high blood pressure.
- Cancer: In 2012, there were approximately 13.7 million Americans with a history of cancer. Some of these men and women were cancer-free and others still had evidence of cancer and could be undergoing treatment. In 2013, there were expected to be 1,660,290 new cancer cases.
- Diabetes: Data from the 2011 National Diabetes Fact Sheet states that 25.8 million people in the United States has diabetes. 1.9 million new adult cases of diabetes were diagnosed in 2010. An update in 2013 states

that the total cost of diagnosed diabetes in the United States in 2012 was $245 billion.

- Osteoporosis: More than 40 million Americans are estimated to already have this disease.

The United States is reported to spend over eight thousand dollars per person on healthcare. It is hard to believe that there are people dying of an inadequate diet in the United States when there is a surplus of food, but it's true. And there appears to be little hope of reversing the trend.

The World Health Organization (WHO) ranked the U.S. number one in health care spending. But even with all this spending, the U.S. ranked 72 in overall health – lower than many Third World countries.

The Real Answer

People like to think that modern medicine is the answer to the health care crisis. But experts in the field of medicine realize that despite the use of advanced technology, there has been no decline in the health crisis.

The real answer does not rely on the curing of disease, but in the prevention of it. And one of the best ways to prevent disease is living a healthy lifestyle. For many people, understanding what constitutes a healthy lifestyle is daunting. Other people know exactly what "healthy living" means, but they are not willing to commit to making the necessary lifestyle changes. Committing to choices like these simply sounds like too much of a hassle:

1. Eat well – Kick the SAD diet out of your life and replace it with a diet filled with fresh fruits and vegetables, whole grains (limited), lean meats, healthy fats, and fish.
2. Exercise well – Exercising just 30 minutes three times per week will promote heart health, help you lose weight by increasing your metabolism, build strong bones, and boost your immune system.

3. Sleep well – Most cell repairs and memory assimilation happen during sleep. Most people need seven to eight hours of sleep each night in order to function at their best.
4. Live well – Believe it or not, kindness and love, as well as having a set of principles to guide your life, will help you to be healthier and live longer.
5. Optimal Nervous System Health – Everything that goes on in our body begins with the nervous system. Ridding your body of blockages in the nervous system, known as subluxations, can help you reach your full potential.

The burden of achieving good health falls squarely on your own shoulders. You cannot rely on others to watch out for your health. You cannot find good health at the doctor's office or in the pharmacy. You can't find it in the junk food aisles of the grocery store or in fast food restaurants. Good health can only be found when you commit to a healthy lifestyle.

By taking care of your body now, learning everything you can to make good choices, and finding practitioners that promote the prevention of disease, you will be well on your way to a healthier you.

CHAPTER 2

The Crisis Care Dilemma

Modern medicine is crisis-focused. It's one of the things that allows the average American to burn the candle at both ends for a few decades, have a little open heart surgery to keep the old ticker chugging along, and skid into a late retirement exhausted, disabled, and broke.

Think about it.

Are you motivated to be well right now, or will you be far more motivated to be well when you get sick and your life is taken away from you? Sadly, we only tend to find our motivation when something goes wrong. It's far easier to choose cheeseburgers and couch time over healthier choices... until all those bad choices finally create a disaster for our health.

That's the real cause of the vast majority of diseases we are dealing with today: lifestyle choices. We should be motivated every day to live a lifestyle that allows us to thrive, maintain, and enjoy a fantastic quality of life. And that's what the wellness movement is all about: seeking wellness instead of seeking cures, each and every day. There is no medication, special lotion, surgery, and injection that re-gains our health back.

Modern medicine runs on the philosophy that aging is the decline phase of life. We are born, we live, we get sick, and we die. But it doesn't have to be that way! There's the first mindset switch we need to make. Instead of thinking of our bodies as vessels destined and designed for deterioration and disease, think of it as being meant for continuous progress. Yes, we will all age, and we will all eventually die. But how would the rest of your life be different if you decided to live up to your physical potential from here on out?

What Is Wellness Care?

More and more people are coming to realize that focusing on their wellness could allow them to live healthier, longer lives. They are demanding that their health care providers work with them on wellness plans that prevent, rather than cure, diseases and pain. There is evidence of this shift all around us:

- Organic and local foods are becoming the preferred produce option in America, and around the world. The USDA's National Farmers Market Directory's listings have increased by more than 61% since 2008.
- The Veterans Administration has committed to implementing alternative therapies to help veterans deal with pain and avoid possible opioid painkiller addictions.
- According to Harvard Medical School, Americans make about 425 million visits to holistic health care providers each year.
- A 2011 Gallup poll showed that half of Americans take vitamins every day.

Part of the wellness revolution has been a shift in the relationship between primary care doctors and patients. By and large, the public no longer chooses to take their doctor's advice as the final word on certain health concerns. We are far more likely today to ask questions, seek second opinions, and research alternative treatments. The patient, rather than the doctor, is now the decision-maker when the patient's wellness is concerned.

What IS Modern Medicine Good For?

Make no mistake: modern medicine still plays an important role in our health care system. And the more open and receptive your primary care physician is to discuss your wellness care, the more of a partner role he or she can play in your ongoing health.

The modern view on health care places all health-related concepts and activities into three categories:

1. Self Care – this includes the choices you make every day about diet, exercise, stress management, and the like.

2. Health Care – this is all of the things you seek help for in order to maintain good health, such as seeking wellness providers, getting educated on fitness and exercise, and taking part in wellness programs physicians are offering.
3. Crisis Care – this is the care we obtain when a disaster strikes; when we get sick or injured, we go to the doctor to help us fix what we cannot handle on our own.

Self care and health care are intended to prevent the need for crisis care. However, choosing to stop smoking will not prevent you from getting into a car accident. There are sure-fire ways to prevent cancer, heart attacks, or other conditions, but of course there are occurrences were serious illnesses, broken bones, failing organs - situations such as these are the rightful domain of crisis care.

A Crash Course in How to Get Well

America's current health care system promotes drugs and surgery above all else – including prevention. Each year, America spends $3 billion on prescription medications and $2 trillion on crisis care. The first tragedy of this situation is that despite all that spending, America is still getting sicker and sicker. The second tragedy is that most of the illnesses for which we seek crisis care are completely preventable.

Chances are, there are about a hundred lifestyle choices you could improve upon. Here are a few simple suggestions to get you back on track:

- Get regular, moderate exercise
- Stay well hydrated
- Eat a plant-based, nutrient-dense diet
- Get adequate sleep
- Quit smoking and any other drug habits
- Enjoy moderate alcohol intake at the most
- Find healthy ways to deal with stress
- Seek activities and people that boost your mood
- Bring aboard health care practitioners you trust to help you feel well

In later chapters, we will dig into many of these topics in more detail. Suffice it to say that people tend to feel stressed and conflicted when making these lifestyle shifts. It's just so much easier to give in to our desires... to be lazy and not hit the gym... to order the cheeseburger because it's on the happy hour menu but the salad isn't... to quit smoking, maybe next week.

All of those choices we make every day seem insignificant in the moment. But it all adds up. In ten, twenty, thirty years from now, will you regret your lifestyle choices? What it all comes down to is this – how can you improve your current level of functioning?

CHAPTER 3

What You Need to Know about Peripheral Neuropathy

What is Peripheral Neuropathy? It helps to break the term down and look at each individual word. **Neuropathy** refers to pain that is caused by nerve damage. The **peripheral** part of the term refers to the peripheral nervous system – that's all of the nerves in your body that radiate out from your spinal cord. So peripheral neuropathy is typically presented as pain and tingling caused by nerve damage in the extremities.

The most common areas affected by peripheral neuropathy are the nerves in the extremities, like your arms, hands, legs, and feet. People with peripheral neuropathy generally describe the pain as stabbing, tingling, numbness, burning, or icy coldness. Many of these patients also report some weakness in the affected area.

Neuropathy of the small fiber nerves reduces sensation and can cause the patient not to be able to feel cuts, burns, punctures, or blisters on the skin. Reduced sensation in the feet can cause car accidents when people fail to sense whether they are pressing the gas pedal or the brake, or they may not be able to regulate the pressure they apply to a pedal.

Neuropathy of the large fiber nerves in the legs can cause loss of balance and coordination. This type of neuropathy causes thousands of falls every year. A fall puts the patient at risk for hip fractures, head traumas, and other serious injuries.

In addition to the extremities, other parts of the body can be affected by neuropathy; for example, the peripheral nervous system also controls your vital organs. Damage to the associated nerves can cause heartburn, indigestion, difficulty swallowing, constipation, and many other problems.

What Causes Peripheral Neuropathy?

Instead of delving into the hundreds of specific causes there are for peripheral neuropathy, we will break them down into three general categories.

1. **Circulation related peripheral neuropathy** is most often experienced by people with diabetes, but anyone with reduced blood circulation is at risk. When the small blood vessels surrounding the nerves die off, the nerves are deprived of nourishment and will also eventually die. The damaged nerves are the source of the pain and tingling. Over 50% of diabetics develop some form of neuropathy (Mayo Clinic). Peripheral neuropathy is also the top cause of amputations for diabetics.
2. **Toxicity related peripheral neuropathy** can be caused by any sort of exposure to toxins.

The two causes we typically focus on are chemotherapy drugs and statins.

a. **Chemotherapy-induced peripheral neuropathy** is a side effect reported by many cancer patients. Some chemotherapy drugs are more likely to cause neuropathy than others. Patients who are on a more frequent treatment schedule are also more likely to experience neuropathy.
b. **Statin-induced peripheral neuropathy** is caused by the use of drugs that doctors prescribe to reduce fats, including triglycerides and cholesterol, in the blood. Instead of prescribing changes in diet and exercise habits to fix the root cause of the cholesterol problem, it is far easier (and more profitable) for a doctor to prescribe a statin.

3. **Trauma induced peripheral neuropathy** is caused by events like car accidents, falls, or athletic injuries. Any of these events can cause damage to the peripheral nerves.

Wearing a cast, walking with crutches, or frequent repetitive motions can also damage nerves. (Mayo Clinic)

One important fact to realize is that regardless of the cause of peripheral neuropathy, the damage is the same under a microscope. The techniques for rebuilding the nerves does not change.

How Do You Treat Peripheral Neuropathy?

Medical doctors routinely tell their patients that nerves cannot regenerate themselves, but it's simply not true! Several treatments have been proven to stimulate the growth of the nerve endings and the blood vessels that nourish them.

If the symptoms are caused by a treatable underlying condition, it is almost always possible to reverse the neuropathy. While medications can reduce the pain associated with peripheral neuropathy, painkillers do nothing to repair or reverse the damage to the nerves and blood vessels. Getting to the root cause of the neuropathy and taking steps to reverse the damage is the only effective and long-lasting method of treatment.

The end goal in treating peripheral neuropathy is to remove blockage so that the nerves can function properly and send and receive messages with the brain. The best way to achieve this is with a comprehensive treatment plan. That's why we use several methods concurrently to treat our peripheral neuropathy patients. At our clinic, peripheral neuropathy appointments last about 45 minutes rather than the standard 15-minute visit.

Peripheral Neuropathy Treatment Options

Low Level Light Therapy (LLLT) – LLLT uses low-power lasers or infrared light-emitting diodes to promote nerve growth, reduce pain, improve immune response, accelerate healing of wounds and fractures, increase collagen and DNA production, and promote fibroblast activity.

Vibration Therapy – Vibration therapy increases balance and mobility, bone density, and range of motion. It also increases blood flow by 15 times.

During vibration therapy, patients sit or stand on a vibrating platform that causes their muscles to contract, increase circulation, as well as nerve stimulation.

ReBuilder System – Uses electrical stimulation of the muscles to improve blood flow and normalize deficits in nerve conduction velocity. The ReBuilder System is trusted by all four Cancer Treatment Centers of America locations to alleviate chemotherapy-induced peripheral neuropathy. Most of their cancer patients who use the Re-Builder System have reduced or stopped taking their pain medicine, as they report drastically reduced pain in their extremities after treatments.

Soft Tissue Therapy - Hand-held soft tissue machines are used to massage the tissue surrounding the areas affected by peripheral neuropathy. Soft tissue therapy targets injured muscles and soft tissue. Massage, pressure, stretching and trigger point techniques are used to promote the restoration of function, improved circulation, and breaking down scar tissue.

Spinal Decompression - When peripheral neuropathy has resulted from an accident or injury that resulted in compressed discs or vertebrae, spinal decompression can provide relief. Spinal decompression is a chiropractic technique that uses traction to take the pressure off the discs and allow the discs to move back into place. It also stimulates blood flow, which produces a healing response.

Traditional chiropractic therapy is used by millions of people to adjust misaligned vertebrae. Regular chiropractic care allows signals to flow between the brain, spinal cord, and nerves. Since chiropractic adjustments promote nervous system function, it should be considered an integral part of any peripheral neuropathy treatment plan. More importantly with neuropathy, chiropractic is used to get the feet and hands more mobile as the neuropathy has created stiffness and mobility problems.

Each intricate part of our program is equally important. Each one relies on the other to do its job. There are a lot of treatments out there that get new blood to the areas temporarily. We know them all; our goal is to repair neuropathy permanently.

These treatment methods will be discussed in more detail in the following chapters.

What Else Can I Do to Reduce My Pain?

There are additional components of a full peripheral neuropathy treatment plan that cannot be controlled in the clinic setting. While we provide our patients with the resources to make the right choices for themselves, it is solely up to them how closely they follow these guidelines.

Nutrition – Committing to dietary changes that reduce inflammation in the body can make a tremendous difference in peripheral neuropathy symptoms. Basically, an anti-inflammatory diet promotes foods that inhibit inflammation (fruits, vegetables, lean omega-3 rich foods) and limits the intake of foods that promote inflammation (sugars, starches, omega-6 foods).

Supplements – Natural Nitric Oxide Boosters is an intricate part of treating peripheral neuropathy. In the following chapters, we will take a closer look at the peripheral neuropathy treatment options we offer in our clinic.

CHAPTER 4

Low Level Light Therapy – Can It Help You?

Since lasers were invented in the 1960's, medical professionals have discovered numerous applications for lasers to improve people's health. Ophthalmologists, dermatologists, and surgeons quickly found lasers to be useful in treating their patients. Low level light therapy (LLLT) is in its fourth decade of use as a method of treating sprains, back and neck pain, arthritis, ulcers, and more.

Looking to the future, studies are currently being conducted to test out LLLT's effectiveness in treating sperm mobility, spinal cord injuries, stroke victims, Parkinson's patients, and Alzheimer's disease.

How Does LLLT Work?

Think back to your high school biology class. You may recall that plants use a process called photosynthesis to produce energy. The plant changes that energy into ATP, which is the fuel stored and used by all cells in all living things – plants and animals alike. LLLT stimulates the production of enzyme cytochrome c oxidase, which, like sunlight for plants, produces ATP. With more fuel being produced, cells have more energy to repair themselves. Currently, numerous studies being conducted around the world are proving that LLLT can help the body regenerate its own tissues, including spinal cord and nerve tissues. The therapy also holds promise for restoring eyesight, reversing numerous neurological diseases, and stroke recovery.

What Else Could LLLT Treat in the Future?

Fibromyalgia is a condition that causes the brain to process pain abnormally, resulting in chronic, widespread pain and chronic fatigue. This condition affects millions of Americans and has been poorly understood and under-diagnosed, resulting in billions of dollars in cost to our health care system.

Fibromyalgia is primarily treated with medications; side effects often make the patient's symptoms even worse. But studies have already shown that LLLT helps to treat the pain and swelling of fibromyalgia.

Parkinson's Disease belongs to a group of conditions called motor system disorders, which are the result of the loss of dopamine-producing brain cells. The four primary symptoms of Parkinson's disease are tremors in the arms, legs, jaw, and face; stiffness of the limbs and trunk; slowness of movement; and impaired balance and coordination.

Many scientists think that one of the malfunctioning systems in Parkinson's disease is located in the mitochondria. These are the cellular systems/organelles that produce ATP, the energy for all the other systems of the body. They also help to detoxify the brain and body by regulating the free radicals circulating in the system.

A study by the UVA Morris K. Udall Parkinson's Research Center of Excellence showed that a single, brief treatment of LLLT increased the movement of the mitochondria in neuron cells to be similar to the level of movement in disease-free, age-matched control groups.

Muscle regeneration is another area where LLLT holds great promise. LLLT has been shown to increase cellular function and regeneration, including cells that create muscle tissue. Studies are being conducted to determine if heart muscles can be regenerated using LLLT.

Medical doctors are taught that heart muscle does not regenerate. Therefore, when someone has a heart attack, doctors tell patients that the muscle that died in the attack is gone for good. However, new research shows that heart muscle can and does regenerate itself. This finding opens up new possibilities of regenerating heart muscle after a heart attack with LLLT, thereby preventing a host of complications including heart failure.

Weight loss might sound like a stretch when you think of the possibilities of LLLT treatment, but it is already being used to help patients achieve their goals. Laser light easily penetrates through layers of skin to activate healing responses within cells and to stimulate nerve endings to produce endorphins. Endorphins, such as serotonin, are produced normally by your body and are nature's natural mood lifter and help prevent you from feeling anxious or moody.

The LLLT therapy of specific points on the body helps to reduce the desire to eat, providing a natural satiation without food. The laser also helps balance organ and glandular functions that regulate weight. Incredibly, LLLT is used in a very similar way to relieve the withdrawal symptoms of quitting smoking!

Diabetic ulcers are one of the many health risks associated with uncontrolled diabetes. Diabetic ulcers are extremely hard to cure. Due to artery abnormalities, diabetic neuropathy, and delayed wound healing, infection or gangrene of the extremities is relatively common.

Wound healing is usually taken care of efficiently by a healthy body. But diabetes is a disorder that impedes normal steps of the wound healing process. Common treatments - skin grafts, moist wound therapy, and negative pressure wound therapy – almost never work completely.

LLLT is a new treatment option for diabetic ulcers that is showing great promise. Unlike other therapies, LLLT has no side effects. In one case study, a man with a diabetic ulcer was treated for a total of 16 sessions of low-intensity laser therapy over a four-week period. During this time, the ulcer healed completely. During a follow-up period of nine months, there was no recurrence of the ulcer.

What Role Does LLLT Play in Treating Peripheral Neuropathy?

Because LLLT stimulates cellular regeneration, it plays a vital role in a complete treatment plan for peripheral neuropathy patients. LLLT helps damaged nerves and their surrounding blood vessels regrow, gradually improving sensation and function for the patient. There are currently no drugs on the market that can help the body heal itself in such a way. Plus, unlike virtually all medications, there are absolutely no side effects associated with LLLT. The area may feel warm or tingly during the treatment, but there are no other reported physical sensations from LLLT patients.

When a patient visits our office for treatment of peripheral neuropathy, we apply LLLT boots around the hands, feet, or both and let the machine deliver the treatment for a specified amount of time.

CHAPTER 5

Electrotherapy for Pain Relief and Nerve Re-education?

Right off the bat, let's get one thing out of the way: this is nothing like the horrifying practice of electroshock therapy that was used in asylums decades ago. And on the other hand, it's more exciting than the electrolysis procedure that can get rid of unwanted body hair.

Electrotherapy is a pain management technique where small electrical currents stimulate nerves and muscles to release pain-killing chemicals such as endorphins, and prevents pain signals from being transmitted to the brain. Electrotherapy also improves nerve function by gently opening up the nerve pathways. It does not hurt your muscles or nerves, and it does not burn your skin. In our office, we rely on the ReBuilder System for patients seeking treatment for peripheral neuropathy. This technology is much different than a TENS unit. TENS units can actually make neuropathy worse over time.

ReBuilder is an FDA-approved device that was designed specifically to treat the pain, burning, numbness, and tingling associated with peripheral neuropathy. In fact, all of the Cancer Treatment Centers of America use ReBuilder to alleviate their patients' chemotherapy-induced neuropathy.

What Are the Benefits of ReBuilder Treatment?

Daily, thirty minute ReBuilder treatments in your home may significantly reduce the amount of pain medications needed to deal with an acute pain syndrome. It has also been used to effectively treat functional problems such as drop foot. The effects of this treatment method are cumulative, meaning that the longer you continue to use it, the better the results you will see.

ReBuilder also increases blood flow, strengthens muscles, and improves the transmission of signals within the nervous system. And when patients experience less pain at night, they tend to get a better night's sleep. This allows them to function better during the daytime and promotes cellular repair and regeneration during their restful hours.

How Do I Use ReBuilder at Home?

You will place small adhesive pads in a supplied footbath, or place the effected areas on specific pads in order to deliver electrical current. Your healthcare provider will help you determine where the pads should be placed for best results. The vast majority of patients, marked improvement in pain, function, and mobility occurs within just a few electrotherapy treatments.

How Does it Work?

All you have to do is put on the pads or garments, turn on the system, and sit back so that the device can do its job. ReBuilder is an "intelligent" system, in that it analyzes the nerves 7.83 times per second, determines the correct amount of electrical signal, and then delivers it to the target area.

The electrical current opens up the nerve pathways and promotes good signal conduction. During treatment, you may feel your muscles contract and relax – this is normal. As you progress through more and more treatments, your condition will improve and the need for electrotherapy is reduced. Throughout the treatment period, the ReBuilder will alter the amount of signal it delivers based on the condition of your nerves.

Whether your peripheral neuropathy is a side effect of statin drugs, chemotherapy treatment, diabetes, or another source, ReBuilder can help restore function and sensation to your peripheral nervous system.

Why Is ReBuilder the Electrotherapy System of Choice?

Since ReBuilder hit the market in the mid 1980's, it has helped millions of patients repair their pain points from the inside out with no drugs, no surgery, and virtually no side effects. When you have dealt with problems like shortness of breath, memory loss, constipation, sleeplessness, and dizziness while on pain medications, the idea of treating the root cause of the pain and eliminating drugs from your daily routine often seems like nothing more than a fantasy. But it's totally possible – perhaps within a week or two – with electrotherapy.

Another benefit of the ReBuilder System is that it shuts off automatically when the treatment time is up. This prevents possible injury, should the patient fall asleep during treatment. ReBuilder also comes with a lifetime warranty.

But the real reason we use ReBuilder for our peripheral neuropathy patients is simple: we have seen the results first-hand. Almost all of our patients who use ReBuilder report feeling less numbness, pain, and tingling in the treated area. With blood flow and nerve function restored, patients become more mobile and stop relying on painkillers to get through the day.

Is ReBuilder Right for Me?

In our clinic, we are all about helping our patients heal from the inside out, without medications or surgery. We use several modalities at once to treat our patients who are suffering from peripheral neuropathy because we believe in a broad-spectrum approach to treating chronic pain. All of the techniques we combine for neuropathy treatment are focused on improving nerve function and regeneration, as well as promoting blood flow.

Our neuropathy patients come to us in the midst of a very difficult period in their lives. They may be going through chemotherapy treatment; maybe they are failing to recover from an automobile accident; they could also be suffering from diabetes-induced neuropathy. While the causes of their pain are different, we use similar methods to treat them all. Electrotherapy is one important treatment method that they all have in common.

Thousands of doctors in all types of practices prescribe the ReBuilder System for their patients. All four Cancer Treatment Centers of America offer it to their patients who are undergoing chemotherapy. And as a matter of fact, using ReBuilder *before* starting treatment can be an effective preventative measure against developing peripheral neuropathy in the first place.

If you are suffering from the effects of peripheral neuropathy, there is an excellent chance that ReBuilder can help. The ReBuilder is only a piece of the puzzle in our innovative program. We strongly believe that a more complete approach to Neuropathy Reveral is a smarter plan of action. That's why we prescribe electrotherapy, low level light therapy, chiropractic, Nutrition, and vibration therapy to our patients who are struggling to get their pain under control and live a active life like they desire.

CHAPTER 6

Soft Tissue Therapy That Keeps You Moving!

Soft tissue therapy includes a variety of massage-type treatments of the soft tissue, which includes muscles, connective tissue, ligaments, and tendons. Soft tissue therapy can effectively treat injuries, pain, and dysfunction.

Soft tissue therapy can help with:

- Carpal tunnel syndrome
- Joint pain
- Shin splints
- Back pain
- Plantar fasciitis
- Fibromyalgia
- Tendinitis

- Groin pulls
- Frozen shoulder

Benefits of Soft Tissue Therapy

Soft tissue therapy is effective in alleviating many symptoms associated with those medical conditions listed above. It can improve the performance of your muscles, circulatory system, joints and immune system. For better range of motion, decreased blood pressure, and to alleviate the pain and stiffness associated with arthritis or fibromyalgia, soft tissue therapy is the drug-free answer you're looking for.

Types of Soft Tissue Therapy

While some soft tissue therapies are delivered by chiropractors, others are offered by massage therapists.

Trigger Point Therapy

Trigger points are those tender "knots" you feel when you or someone rubs a sore spot. Your chiropractor will apply pressure to trigger points to relieve pain and dysfunction in other parts of the body – this is called trigger point therapy.

There are two basic types of trigger points: active and latent.

- Active trigger points cause muscular pain and transfer pain to other areas of the body when your chiropractor applies pressure. For example, pressing on a trigger point between your shoulders may send shooting pain down your arm.
- Latent trigger points do not refer pain to other areas of the body, and cause stiffness in the joints and restricted range of motion.

Trigger points develop due to several causes, including birth trauma, an injury sustained in a fall or accident, poor posture, or overexertion.

After several treatments of trigger point therapy, the swelling and stiffness of muscular pain is reduced, range of motion is increased, tension is relieved, and circulation, flexibility and coordination are improved.

Swedish Massage

Swedish massage is the most common type of massage in the United States. In Swedish massage, your massage therapist will lubricate the skin with massage oil and use various strokes, like gliding, kneading, friction, stretching and tapping, to warm up and work the muscle tissue. This helps to release tension and break up muscle knots. This mode of treatment helps to reduce swelling and inflammation, as well as promote relaxation.

Cross Friction Massage

Soft tissues can become stressed beyond their limits, resulting in small, microscopic tears. When these tears occur, the body responds by causing inflammation, which helps in the role of healing. However, too much inflammation can form scar tissue.

Continuing to use the muscle as it is torn can increase the chance of more scarring. Scar tissue is tough and decreases mobility and elasticity. This results in loss of function, resulting in more tearing and inflammation, resulting in more scar tissue... a vicious cycle.

For cross friction massage, your massage therapist will apply his fingers directly over the tissue involved. The key here is for the massage to be opposite the direction of the tissue fibers. This "transverse friction" massage keeps adhesions and scar tissue from forming. It also results in improved range of motion and less pain.

Cross friction massage is a highly effective treatment for injuries to the muscles, tendons, and ligaments caused by micro-tears. Cross friction creates heat, which helps to mobilize adhesions (bands of scar tissue) between fascial layers, muscles, and other soft tissues. This heat helps to promote healing.

Knee injuries are extremely common, but the healing process can be quite frustrating. In a 2009 study, bilateral knee injuries were treated with cross friction massage one week following injury. Fifty-one participants received between nine and 30 treatments. After four weeks of cross friction massage, the knees were stronger, less stiff and could absorb more energy.

Myofascial Release Therapy

Myofascial release is a stretching technique used by chiropractors to treat soft tissue problems. To understand what it is and how it works, you first need to know a few things about fascia.

Fascia is a thin tissue that covers the muscles and every fiber within each muscle. This means that when you stretch your muscles, you are really stretching your muscles and your fascia.

When muscle fibers are injured, the fibers and the fascia surrounding it become short and tight. This uneven stress can cause pain and other symptoms. Myofascial release treats these symptoms by releasing the uneven tightness in injured fascia.

The stretching is determined by your chiropractor as he feels what each stretch does to your body. The feedback he receives helps him decide how much force to use, the direction of the stretch, and how long to stretch.

Your chiropractor will find areas of tightness and then apply a light stretch. Once your muscle and fascia have relaxed, he will increase the stretch. This process is repeated until the area is fully relaxed. Then, the next affected area is stretched.

One area that myofascial release therapy holds great promise is in the treatment of scoliosis, which is an abnormal curvature of the spine. A 2008 case study of an 18-year-old female subject observed her progress as she underwent six weeks of myofascial release therapy. The subject received treatment consisting of two sessions each week for 60 minutes. Pain, pulmonary function and quality of life were measured at predetermined intervals. The subject improved with pain levels, trunk rotation, posture, quality of life, and pulmonary function.

Active Release Therapy (ART)

One goal of Active Release Therapy (ART) is to restore normal texture, motion, and function of soft tissues. Another goal is to release any trapped nerves or blood vessels. This is accomplished through the removal of adhesions as your chiropractor applies stretching and massage techniques.

Adhesions happen for two reasons. One reason is acute injury, such as a blow, fall, pull, or strain. The second reason is repetitive overuse, which can happen with improper posture, compensating for injuries (i.e. limping), or repetitive motions. The result is that the area is compressed and tissues suffer from decreased blood supply. The soft tissues respond by forming scar tissue. This results in pain, poor mobility, and a continued injury cycle.

Your chiropractor will determine which soft tissue is affected. Then specific massage techniques are used to make these tissues slide over one another with a hand, finger, or thumb.

In the first three levels of ART treatment, all movement is facilitated by your chiropractor. In level four of the treatment, your chiropractor will have you move in specific ways as he applies pressure.

ART is a great treatment option for carpal tunnel syndrome, sciatica, TMJ, and other problems.

Muscle Energy Technique (MET)

Muscle energy technique (MET) is based on the idea that muscles on one side of a joint relax as the other side of the joint contracts.

MET is used to:

- Lengthen shortened or spastic muscles
- Improve weakened ligaments and muscle strength
- Improve range of motion

During an MET treatment, your chiropractor will ask you to contract a muscle for approximately five seconds while he applies an anti-force to that muscle. Each time you contract your muscle, it stretches further. Muscle energy techniques can be applied safely to almost any joint in the body.

Graston Technique

The Graston Technique helps your chiropractor break up scar tissue. This technique uses specially designed instruments to identify and treat areas exhibiting soft tissue issues. The edges of the tools mold to the various shapes of the body.

The Graston tools act like tuning fork instruments, vibrating in your chiropractor's hand. This allows him to find specific adhesions and restrictions, and treat them very precisely. Deeper adhesions can be treated with Graston tools than without them.

Which type of soft tissue therapy is right for you? Our team will evaluate what type of muscle work you may need. They will administer the appropriate treatments available when you go in for your evaluation. These treatments often work together to provide better circulation, pain relief and range of motion in a shorter amount of time than either modality can deliver on its own.

CHAPTER 7

Surprising Relief Comes from Vibration Therapy

Health care providers, physical therapists, chiropractors, and personal trainers use whole body vibration therapy (WBVT), for a surprisingly wide range of purposes. Specifically, vibration therapy is great for:

- Increasing muscle endurance, coordination, and strength
- Better circulation of lymph fluid and blood for better healing, energy, and overall health
- Improving nerve activity
- Boosting bone density and fighting off osteoporosis

For our patients with peripheral neuropathy, vibration therapy reduces their pain, increases circulation, improves strength and flexibility, and increases energy, mobility, and balance. We achieve these results without drugs or invasive surgery.

A recent study showed that patients with diabetic peripheral neuropathy (DPN) specifically have much to gain from vibration therapy. Study participants were observed to determine how effective whole body vibration therapy really is in treating pain associated with DPN. The study's participants received three whole body vibration treatments per week for a month. Each session consisted of four rounds of three minutes of vibration. The study's results demonstrated significant pain reduction overall, and no side-effects were observed during the study.

WBVT allows individuals to experience less pain without invasive surgery, and usually reduces or even eliminates the need for pain medication. The high-frequency vertical vibrations produced by the device assist in increasing circulation, rebuilding muscle tissue, improving range of motion, and reducing pain and stress. But the benefits go even further beyond getting off pain medications. Patients are likely to see far fewer serious injuries and infections due to increased sensation and better coordination. And diabetics in particular will be at lower risk of limb amputation due to reduced infection rates.

How Does WBVT Work?

Vibration therapy devices come in a range of forms. There are vibrating foot platforms that treat just peripheral neuropathy of the feet. Some practitioners use hand-held devices to target very specific areas of the body and fully customize the length and duration of treatment. Other health care providers prefer vibrating chairs or platforms that patients may sit or stand on for a full-body treatment. Either way, the high frequency vibration is an effective and safe treatment for the area(s) of the body affected by neuropathy.

Vibration therapy stimulates a patient's muscles to rapidly contract. Frequent tightening of a muscle will build and strengthen the muscle tissue, even when it's performed for small bits of time. As the muscle builds, its need for blood also grows. This is what stimulates blood vessels to grow and keep fueling the muscles with the nutrients they need during and after vibration therapy.

It's important to note that while traditional exercise is difficult and often uncomfortable for many patients dealing with chronic pain, vibration therapy cuts these complications out of the equation. When people have reduced sensation in their feet and hands, it can be downright dangerous to pick up free weights or hop onto a treadmill. But vibration therapy allows the patient to sit down throughout the "workout," even though muscles are being strengthened the entire time.

When the muscles are pushed and exerted in specific ways, the nerves can be stimulated to regrow their neural pathways and even repair or rebuild the damaged nerves.

An added bonus of vibration therapy is that it stimulates the release of osteoblasts from the nuclei in bone cells. Osteoblasts are what make it possible for bones to grow stronger by creating new bone cells.

All of these facts combined means that vibration therapy patients will regain sensation, strength, and stamina. Over time, the little things in life that used to be exhausting will become far easier. Eventually, patients get back to more normal routines and introduce regular moderate exercise to their daily calendars. It is truly an eye-opening experience to lose full use of parts of your body, and then gain it back again. Your priorities and your perspective will never be the same.

Is There Anybody Who Should NOT Experience WBVT?

Certain patients should not participate in vibration therapy, including patients with epilepsy, severe vertigo, or a detached retina. Also, if you are pregnant, vibration therapy is probably not safe for you.

For the rest of our patients who may benefit from it, we recommend vibration therapy, which we also provide in our office. Vibration therapy treatments usually last no more than about 15 minutes. But the key to effectively treating many conditions, including peripheral neuropathy, is to approach it with several different modalities. That's why we never treat a PN patient with just vibration therapy.

Our PN patients commonly experience vibration therapy, low-level light therapy, soft tissue treatments, electrical stimulation, and a chiropractic adjustment during their visits. We go at these pain-related conditions with everything we've got, because patient comfort, health, and satisfaction is paramount. We know that this multi-pronged approach is the best way to get people off painkillers and back on their feet. That's why we also continuously counsel our patients about the importance of proper hydration and diet. You really are what you eat, so it's crucial to fuel your body with healthy, high-quality foods that will promote growth, healing, and wellness in every cell of your body. Continue on to the next chapter to learn more about the role good nutrition plays in your recovery from peripheral neuropathy.

CHAPTER 8

Good Health Starts with Good Nutrition

Getting regular exercise, dealing with stress in healthy ways, and eating a diet rich in plant-based whole foods is a great start toward achieving good health. But no matter how well you stick to these tips, you are always at risk for your body to be damaged at the cellular level. Environmental factors play a huge part in this damage by introducing free radicals into our bodies.

What Are Free Radicals?

Free radicals form in the human body when an electron in an atom becomes unpaired and searches for another electron to pair with. It may sounds like an insignificant event, but this search for another unpaired atom causes damage to our cells and a chain reaction of more free radical creation.

Daily life exposes us to free radicals all the time, from the foods we eat and the air we breathe. Free radicals cause illness and contribute to the aging process. They have a negative impact on how we look and feel. Free radicals occur in everyday life but are made worse by:

- Eating a diet full of processed foods and produce treated with chemicals
- Smoking
- Using drugs
- Failure to deal correctly with stress
- Excessive sun exposure
- Pollution

Free radical damage can lead to:

- Cancer
- Heart Disease
- Diabetes

- Arthritis
- Autoimmune diseases

One thing we can do to fight free radicals is to get more antioxidants in our diets. Antioxidants are vitamins, minerals, and other nutrients that protect the body and fight off free radicals. They give free radicals an electron to pair with before the stray electrons can damage our cells. Some examples of antioxidants are beta carotene, vitamin C, and vitamin E. These vitamins help strengthen the immune system, too. Plus, they're readily available in many plant-based foods which we should consume more of, anyway!

Beta Carotene

Beta carotene is one of a group of red, orange, and yellow pigments called carotenoids. Beta carotene and other carotenoids provide approximately 50% of the Vitamin A needed in our daily diet.

Beta carotene is a substance the body converts into Vitamin A. It's a powerful antioxidant that also helps protect the cells and boost the immune system. Sources of this important nutrient include:

- Carrots
- Pumpkins
- Sweet Potatoes
- Spinach
- Collards
- Kale
- Turnip greens
- Beet greens
- Winter squash
- Cabbage

If you would rather get your vitamin A straight-up instead of through the beta carotene conversion, eat more:

- Beef
- Broccoli
- Cantaloupe
- Apricots
- Liver
- Milk
- Butter

- Cheese
- Whole eggs

Vitamin C

When your mom told you to drink orange juice to get over a cold faster, she was right! Vitamin C is another antioxidant that strengthens the immune system. It's vital to the growth and repair of skin, blood vessels, ligaments, and tendons. It is also involved with healing wounds and forming scar tissue.

Plus, vitamin C is important for the formation of collagen, which holds your body's cells together. And, it plays an important role in maintaining oral and eye health.

Many fruits are excellent sources of vitamin C, including:

- Cantaloupe
- Citrus fruits
- Kiwi
- Mango
- Guava

- Papaya
- Pineapple
- Berries
- Watermelon

You can get vitamin C from vegetables too, like cruciferous veggies (broccoli, cauliflower, and Brussels sprouts), peppers, leafy greens, potatoes, tomatoes, and squash.

Vitamin E

The third antioxidant we're concerned about is vitamin E. This nutrient helps widen blood vessels and keeps blood from clotting inside them. Foods that are high in vitamin E will also protect your skin from ultraviolet light, which is a major cause of free radical formation in the body.

Excellent sources of vitamin E include:

- Spinach
- Chard
- Turnip greens
- Mustard greens
- Cayenne pepper

- Asparagus
- Bell peppers
- Eggs
- Nuts and seeds
- Meats
- Olive oil
- Whole grains

Nutrition

Eating a well-balanced diet should provide essential nutrients, but there are some situations that definitely call for adding in supplements. When your diet isn't properly balanced, it doesn't contain adequate amounts of certain nutrients. In this case, supplements may be absolutely necessary.

In order for our body to use food to repair and create cells and tissues, it needs the proper tools. The following nutrients are extremely important to maintain a healthy body. And just like the majority of antioxidant sources, these nutrients are often found in abundance in plant-sourced foods.

Magnesium is not only an essential nutrient, but is responsible for a vast variety of healthy body functions. It also is the most deficient mineral in the Standard American Diet because it can be difficult to meet the daily requirements just from food. Less than 30% of U.S. adults consume the Recommended Daily Allowance of magnesium. And nearly 20% get only half of the magnesium they need daily to remain healthy.

To make sure you get enough magnesium in your diet, eat plenty of whole grains, legumes, vegetables, nuts, seeds, and seafood.

Calcium is the most abundant mineral in your body. It is responsible for strong teeth and bones, as well as proper function of blood vessels, nerve communication, and muscles. Many Americans suffer from a deficiency in calcium. We lose calcium each day through our skin, nails, hair, sweat, and waste.

To make sure you get enough calcium in your diet, make sure you consume dairy products, broccoli, kale, Chinese cabbage, and salmon regularly. Depending on your diet and age, your doctor might recommend a calcium supplement.

Iron is important for the production of hemoglobin (found in red blood cells) and myoglobin (found in muscles). These proteins carry and store oxygen throughout the body. When you don't have enough iron in your body you feel tired, weak, and unable to focus. Few people ever have too much iron in the body, but this rare condition is toxic.

Excellent sources of iron include red meat, liver, egg yolks, leafy green veggies, dried fruits, shellfish, beans, lentils, and artichokes. Pairing iron-rich foods with vitamin C-rich foods will help your body absorb the iron better.

Iron deficiency can affect anyone, but it is extremely common among women of childbearing age. Your chiropractor can help you adjust your diet or recommend an iron supplement when necessary.

Vitamin D helps our bodies in the absorption of calcium. Vitamin D also increases bone density and helps prevent bone fractures. Plus, calcium helps regulate the immune system and protects against some types of cancer.

Humans can synthesize their own vitamin D – all it takes is a little sunshine. If you spend a little time in the sun each day, it is unlikely you will be deficient in vitamin D.

People in warm climates rarely have vitamin D problems – it's our neighbors to the north who tend to hibernate through cold, cloudy winters who suffer. If you live far north of the equator, all it really takes is exposing your skin to the sun for about 20 minutes per day (or a little bit longer for older or dark-skinned people) prior to applying sunscreen on most summer days. If you do this, your body will probably synthesize enough vitamin D to last the whole year.

Folic acid is a B vitamin. It helps your body make new cells, repair DNA, and prevent Alzheimer's, anemia, and some forms of cancer.

It is extremely important for pregnant women to get enough folic acid not only while pregnant, but prior to pregnancy too. One of the first stages of pregnancy includes the development of the brain and spinal cord, so getting enough folic acid during this process is vital to proper fetal development. Insufficient folic acid has been linked to birth defects including spina bifida and anencephaly.

Veggies and citrus fruits are the best sources of folic acid. Eat plenty of dark leafy greens, asparagus, broccoli, beans, citrus fruits, peas, lentils, avocado, seeds and nuts, carrots, and squash.

Eating a healthy, well-balanced diet can provide you with a strong, energetic, efficient, healthy body. The best way to know if you are getting all the elements that make up a fully functioning healthy body is to discuss your diet with your chiropractor or health care professional. Together, you can ensure that you are providing the optimum fuel to your body.

Your body is designed to heal itself. The nervous system is what controls your immune system. If you're run down, your body is less able to cope with germs and infections. This is when we tend to experience illness or pain. If your nervous system is strong and healthy, your body can deal with injuries and germs better. Chiropractic care focuses on helping you maintain a strong and healthy nervous system, resulting in a healthy body and lifestyle.

CHAPTER 9

Getting Back to the Basics of Wellness

For a moment, think back to when you were a kid. Chances are that back in elementary school, you had boundless energy. The days were long but it didn't matter - you could probably run around the neighborhood with your friends with hardly a thought of food, pain, or fatigue.

Now maybe you have kids or grandkids, and you watch them go at playtime for hours without a pause – and it's exhausting! We joke about bottling all that energy. We get nostalgic about feeling limitless and free, but not enough of us know that there really is a way to regain some of those powerful feelings again.

Wellness is very personal and means different things to different people in terms of preferences and outcomes.

- If you have debilitating back pain, you might feel powerful again if you could get through the day without taking prescription painkillers and suffering through their side effects.
- If your arthritis restricts your daily physical activities, you might feel powerful again if you could go for a hike again, or knit another afghan without it resulting in days of excruciating joint pain.
- If you suffer from peripheral neuropathy, you might feel powerful again if you could regain sensation in your fingertips again and take up the activities and hobbies you left behind years ago.

Getting older isn't for sissies – but remember that we are lucky to have made it this far!

So what will it take for you to feel energetic and powerful again? There is no correct blanket answer to that question. Every person presents their own set of symptoms, conditions, and preferences. Plus, each person has their own set of goals that will make them feel healthy and happy. All of that makes it complicated to prescribe a roadmap to wellness.

As we discussed in prior chapters, we offer several healing modalities in our office that patients with chronic pain find to be beneficial. Vibration, low-light laser therapy, and electro therapy are a few important resources that many of our patients use every day. We also counsel our patients about the importance of eating a well-balanced diet.

Good nutrition should be considered the cornerstone of any wellness plan. The food you use to fuel your body will make a huge difference when your cells need to repair and regenerate themselves. We promote a diet that's big on unprocessed foods, fruits, vegetables, whole grains, and lean protein. Eating like this gives your body the vitamins, minerals, and antioxidants it needs to stay strong and healthy.

What Else Can I Do to Feel Well?

At the heart of our practice is a busy wellness clinic that offers chiropractic. We strongly believe in the power of a strong, aligned spine that supports a healthy central nervous system. Keeping the spine aligned is achieved through gentle, routine chiropractic adjustments. For most of our patients, one adjustment a week works great. But patients recovering from an accident, illness, infection, or injury sometimes require more frequent adjustments for a period of time.

Regular chiropractic adjustments can not only improve the health of your spine and nervous system, but they can also:

- Improve mood
- Improve sleep
- Increase energy
- Decrease pain
- Boost flexibility and mobility
- Stop recurring headaches

One of the most important things chiropractic adjustments do is boost the immune system. This is accomplished by clearing the neural pathways so that the central nervous system can communicate effectively with the immune system (and every other system in your body). This communication is hindered when the spine experiences subluxations, which are misalignments along the spinal column. When the nervous system's pathways are cleared, the effects can be quite powerful:

- Decrease in colds, flu, and other contagious illnesses
- Slash the symptoms of asthma and allergies
- Result in fewer hospital admissions

Unfortunately, most people only think to go to the chiropractor if their back hurts. But we can do so much more together than just fix back pain!

What Does Chiropractic Do for Peripheral Neuropathy?

As you may recall, the treatment modalities we already discussed for peripheral neuropathy were all about rebuilding nerves, growing blood vessels, and improving muscle function. Well chiropractic is all about clearing the way for the nervous system to do its job right. So when your brain can tell those tiny nerve endings that it's time to regrow, all those other efforts we talked about are far more likely to be successful.

In addition to fostering the regrowth of damaged nerves, chiropractic can also un-pinch nerves. A pinched nerve can cause numbness and pain, just like peripheral neuropathy. Getting the bones back into their proper places takes pressure off nerves, alleviates pain, and promotes a healthy, active lifestyle. It also gets the joint in the hands, feet or both moving better if affected by neuropathy.

What Should I Do if I Suspect That I Have Peripheral Neuropathy?

The National Institutes of Neurological Disorders and Stroke says that peripheral neuropathy affects roughly 24 million Americans. It's a very common condition among people in certain populations, such as diabetics, cancer patients, and those taking statin medications to lower their cholesterol. Therefore, it's important to know that if you do have peripheral neuropathy, you are certainly not alone.

While the early stages of the symptoms may seem to be just minor irritations, early diagnosis of peripheral neuropathy can prevent the condition from becoming worse. Talk to your doctor right away to diagnose and determine the cause of your peripheral neuropathy. There could be ways to change your medical treatment plan that can reduce your symptoms.

We also strongly recommend visiting your BluePrint To Healthcare as soon as you can. They may be able to offer you a variety of treatments that can reduce or even eliminate the pain, numbness, and tingling associated with PN. There is no reason to wait until the problem becomes worse – as soon as you suspect that something is wrong, seek professional help. It's the best way to ensure your health and wellness for many years to come.

CHAPTER 10

Testimonials

"After 31 visits, I was 90-95% cured & I am very fortunate that I came to Blueprint to Healthcare."

–Bill M.

"After only 2 treatments I was able to sleep at night without socks which had been one of my big problems because my feet had been so cold."

–Mickey W.

"I was taking pain medication every day, after 12 visits I stopped taking pain medication. I had no symptoms at night and I did not need sleeping aids anymore. I am extremely happy with my choice to begin the program."

–Rosanna V.

"I have gone from 44% sensory loss down to 15% sensory loss halfway through the program. I'm getting better and I feel a whole lot better."

–Kim M.

"I saw an ad for neuropathy which intrigued me because I was developing neuropathy in my feet and legs. I saw my podiatrist and he confirmed that I have neuropathy. So, I decided to try the program; I had always had trouble with my legs particularly. I could not sleep at night because my legs bothered me so much – in less than 2 weeks I was beginning to sleep through the night!"

–Bob B.

“I came here because of the numbness in my feet, it was all over the top and bottom of my feet as well as my toes. I’ve been on the program awhile now and all I have is a little bit of numbness so it is definitely working. I would encourage anyone to come here and visit with them. I have been very happy and I believe their maintenance program will help me as well!”

–Matt B.

“Over 5 years ago, I was told by a well-respected neurologist that “nothing can be done other than take B12 and be careful not to fall”. I heard about this program at a local rotary meeting, thought I would give it a try...fully expecting a similar situation because of my age. To my surprise after testing, I knew there was potential that I could really get some help. I am now in my 8th week of therapy and the results have been amazing. No longer have tingling sensation or pain.”

–Burnell S.

"I have been coming to Blueprint to Healthcare for about a week and half now. Since then I have lost nine pounds sticking to the nutrition plan. I have such bad feet problems, back pain, neck pain, and hand pain that's why I decided to come... since I've been coming, I have already seen quite a bit of difference in this short amount of time. I can't believe the progress I've had in such a short amount of time."

–Ann R.

"My feet have been dead for quite some time. Two different times in my pick-up, I couldn't feel my accelerator. We started the treatment and about 3-4 weeks into the program, after beginning the home treatment...I could feel the carpet when I was walking and that was the first time I had done that in quite some time."

–Mark O.

"I was having pretty bad neuropathy and it was continuing to get worse after seeing medical doctors, they were just giving me some pain pills and vitamin B12 shots. I decided I needed to do something better & be proactive. This will be my third week and between all the treatments they do here, I am already improving – I'm down to one incident a week and I was having 5-6 incidents a day."

–Kelly C.

"Neuropathy was effecting my life pretty bad for almost a year now, to the point where I was in pain most of the time. Since I've been coming here for 3 or 4 sessions now, I have already noticed a lot of difference and I am already feeling a lot better.

–Jesse R.

"I came here very apprehensive. I have been coming only a few weeks now and I have already regained so much strength in my left leg which was the problem. I barely use my cane at all now

– just for a little security. I just can't believe how well I am doing after only being treated for a short amount of time!"

–Dorothy C.

"I have suffered from neuropathy for at least three years, I have been completing treatment here and it has already been successful. I can sleep at night without my feet burning and hurting!"

–Betty P.

"I came to Blueprint to Neuropathy because I have neuropathy and it is effecting my golf game. I have been coming about five weeks and I can already tell some improvement in the bottom of my feet."

–Gary C.

"I am relatively new to the program, this is only my third visit. I have already gone from a pain level of 8 to a pain level of 2!"

– Kim N.

"I have been coming about 6 weeks. When I came in, I had severe pain all the way from my hip down to my big toe. As of today, I am able to wiggle my big toe and I have feeling in it! I have NO more pain in my hips or legs. Overall, my time spent here has been well worthwhile! I must say that the staff has been very professional, helpful, and encouraging."

–Nell M.

"I am in my 3rd week of my treatment, when I came in, my left foot was killing me and my right foot was not far behind it. I was asked to rate my pain on a level of 1 – 10 during my consultation and I have been at a level 10 for about three or four months now. My pain level now is nearly gone completely."

–James F.

"I came here after seeing the ad in the paper, I decided to come in because of my neuropathy being so bad. It took a little bit of work but everything they have done here for me has been very great. The staff here is very nice which helps a lot when coming in for treatment."

–Everisto M.

Bibliography

1. Go AS, Mozaffarian D, Roger VL, Benjamin EJ, Berry JD, Borden WB, Bravata DM, Dai S, Ford ES, Fox CS, Franco S, Fullerton HJ, Gillespie C, Hailpern SM, Heit JA, Howard VJ, Huffman MD, Kissela BM, Kittner SJ, Lackland DT, Lichtman JH, Lisabeth LD, Magid D, Marcus GM, Marelli A, Matchar DB, McGuire DK, Mohler ER, Moy CS, Mussolino ME, Nichol G, Paynter NP, Schreiner PJ, Sorlie PD, Stein J, Turan TN, Virani SS, Wong ND, Woo D, Turner MB; on behalf of the American Heart Association Statistics Committee and Stroke Statistics Subcommittee. Heart disease and stroke statistics—2013 update: a

report from the American Heart Association. Circulation.2013;127:e6-e245.

2. Masters, Ryan, PhD. News. Columbia University Mailman School of Public Health. "Obesity Kills More Americans Than Previously Thought". N.p., 15 Aug. 2013.
3. Kochanek KD, Xu JQ, Murphy SL, Miniño AM, Kung HC. Deaths: final data for 2009. Adobe PDF file [PDF-2M] National vital statistics reports. 2011; 60(3).
4. Heidenreich PA, Trogdon JG, Khavjou OA, et al. Forecasting the future of cardiovascular disease in the United States: a policy statement from the American Heart Association. Circulation. 2011;123:933-44. Epub 2011 Jan 24.
5. Go AS, Mozaffarian D, Roger VL, Benjamin EJ, Berry JD, Borden WB, Bravata DM, Dai S, Ford ES, Fox CS, Franco S, Fullerton HJ, Gillespie C, Hailpern SM, Heit JA, Howard VJ, Huffman MD, Kissela BM, Kittner SJ, Lackland DT, Lichtman JH, Lisabeth LD, Magid D,

Marcus GM, Marelli A, Matchar DB, McGuire DK, Mohler ER, Moy CS, Mussolino ME, Nichol G, Paynter NP, Schreiner PJ, Sorlie PD, Stein J, Turan TN, Virani SS, Wong ND, Woo D, Turner MB; on behalf of the American Heart Association Statistics Committee and Stroke Statistics Subcommittee. Heart disease and stroke statistics—2013 update: a report from the American Heart Association. Circulation.2013;127:e6-e245.

6. Go AS, Mozaffarian D, Roger VL, Benjamin EJ, Berry JD, Borden WB, Bravata DM, Dai S, Ford ES, Fox CS, Franco S, Fullerton HJ, Gillespie C, Hailpern SM, Heit JA, Howard VJ, Huffman MD, Kissela BM, Kittner SJ, Lackland DT, Lichtman JH, Lisabeth LD, Magid D, Marcus GM, Marelli A, Matchar DB, McGuire DK, Mohler ER, Moy CS, Mussolino ME, Nichol G, Paynter NP, Schreiner PJ, Sorlie PD, Stein J, Turan TN, Virani SS, Wong ND, Woo D, Turner MB; on behalf of the American Heart Association Statistics Committee and Stroke Statistics Subcommittee. Heart

disease and stroke statistics—2013 update: a report from the American Heart Association. Circulation.2013;127:e6-e245.

7. American Cancer Society. Cancer Facts & Figures 2013. Atlanta: American Cancer Society; 2013.
8. "Diabetes Statistics." Diabetes Basics. American Diabetes Association, 2013.
9. "Osteoporosis." NIHSeniorHealth.
10. Chris L. Peterson, Rachel Burton. The U.S. Health Care Spending. 2008.
11. Kane, Jason. "Health Costs: How the U.S. Compares With Other Countries." PBS. PBS, 22 Oct. 2012. Web.
12. "News Release." USDA Celebrates National Farmers Market Week, August 4-10. United States Department of Agriculture, 5 Aug. 2013. Web. 02 Aug. 2015. <http://www.usda.gov/wps/portal/usda/usdahome?contentid=2013%2F08%2F0155.xml>.

13. "Office of Public and Intergovernmental Affairs." News Releases -. VA Office of Public and Intergovernmental Affairs, 25 Feb. 2014. Web. 02 Aug. 2015. <http://www.va.gov/opa/pressrel/pressrelease.cfm?id=2529>.

14. Eisenberg, DM, Kessler, RC, et al. New England Journal Medicine, "Unconventional Medicine in the United States -- Prevalence, Costs, and Patterns of Use." 1993.

15. Swift, Art. "Half of Americans Take Vitamins Regularly." Gallup.com. N.p., 19 Dec. 2013. Web. 02 Aug. 2015. <http://www.gallup.com/poll/166541/half-americans-vitamins-regularly.aspx>.

16. Who Killed Health Care?: America's $2 Trillion Medical Problem - and the Consumer-Driven Cure, Regina Herzlinger, 2007.

17. Mayo Clinic Staff. "Peripheral Neuropathy." Causes. Mayo Clinic, 04 Dec. 2014. Web. 22 July 2015. http://www.mayoclinic.org/diseases-conditions/peripheral-neuropathy/basics/causes/CON-20019948.

18. “The ReBuilder® Stops Pain While Treating Your Nerves - at Home.” Safe, Effective Neuropathy Treatment. Web. 25 July 2015. <http://www.rebuildermedical.com/>.

19. “Frequently Asked Questions.” Frequently Asked Questions. Web. 25 July 2015. <http://www.rebuildermedical.com/frequently-asked-questions.php#chemo>.

20. Loghmani MT, Warden SJ. “Instrument-assisted cross-fiber massage accelerates knee ligament healing.” Journal of Orthopaedic Sports Physical Therapy. 2009.

21. LeBauer A, Brtalik R, Stowe K. “The effect of myofascial release (MFR) on an adult with idiopathic scoliosis.” Journal of Bodywork and Movement Therapies. 2008.

22. J Bodyw Mov Ther. 2013 Oct;17(4):518-22. doi: 10.1016/j.jbmt.2013.03.001. Epub 2013 Apr 30. http://www.ncbi.nlm.nih.gov/pubmed/24139013.

23. “Why Use VibePlate for Vibration Therapy, Vibration Traning, & Vibration Exercise.”

Why Use VibePlate for Vibration Therapy, Vibration Traning, & Vibration Exercise. N.p., n.d. Web. 26 July 2015. <http://www.vibeplate.net/why-vibeplate>.

24. MedlinePlus (June 7, 2012). U.S. National Library of Medicine. Medline Plus Trusted Health Information for You. Beta-carotene. Retrieved from www.nlm.nih.gov/medlineplus/druginfo/natural/999.html.

25. LL Magnetic Clay Inc.(1996-2010). Ancient Minerals:.Need More Magnesium? 10 Signs to Watch For. Retrieved from: www.ancient-minerals.com/magnesium-deficiency/need-more/.

26. WebMD.(2005–2012). Weight Loss & Diet Plans. Top 10 Iron-Rich Foods. Retrieved from: www.webmd.com/diet/features/top-10-iron-rich-foods.

27. More, J. (Sept. 2008). The British Dietetic Association. Vitamin D- The Unique Vitamin. Retrieved from: www.bda.uk.com/foodfacts/VitaminD.pdf.

28. Ferreira, Leonor Mateus. "Chiropractic Care May Help Control Peripheral Neuropathy in Diabetics." Diabetes News Journal. N.p., 16 Mar. 2015. Web. 27 July 2015. <http://diabetesnewsjournal.com/2015/03/17/chiropractic-care-may-help-control-peripheral-neuropathy-in-diabetics/>.

Notes

Notes

Notes

Notes

Notes

Notes

Notes

Made in the USA
Middletown, DE
16 February 2024

49304006R00066